Juicing for Weight Loss

A Quick Guide to Help You Lose Weight, Detox Body and Boost Energy

Sarah Sparrow

PUBLISHED BY:
Sarah Sparrow
Copyright © 2012

Disclaimer
The information contained in this book is for general information purposes only. The information is provided by the authors and while we endeavor to keep the information up to date and correct, we make no representations or warranties of any kind, express or implied, about the completeness, accuracy, reliability, suitability or availability with respect to the book or the information, products, services, or related graphics contained in the book for any purpose. Any reliance you place on such information is therefore strictly at your own risk.

Table of Contents

Chapter 1: Introduction 4

What is Juicing? 5

Why Do the Juice Diet? 5

Understanding Juice Fasting 5

Understanding Detox Diet 6

Effective Weight Loss through Juicing 7

Goodbye Vitamins and Supplements! 8

How Long Does It Take To Lose Weight On a Juice Diet? 9

Chapter 2: Nutritional Benefits of Juicing 9

Benefits of Juicing 10

Four Benefits of Juicing Raw Fruits 12

Four Benefits of Juicing Raw Vegetables 13

Preventing Diseases through Juicing 14

Micronutrients in Fruits and Vegetables That Enhance Weight Loss
.... 15

Five Major Advantages of Juicing Over Eating Whole Fruits and
Vegetables 17

Chapter 3: The Side Effects of Juicing 18

Low Fiber, Protein and Fat Intake during a Juice Diet: Cons 22

Not Losing Weight When on a Juice Diet 23

Chapter 4: Effective Fasting for Weight Loss 26

Before You Begin 26

Beginning the Fast: When and How? 27

How Long Should a Juice Fast Last? 28

Top Ten Tips for Effective Fasting 28

Eating Solids during a Juice Fast 29

Taking Antidepressants on a Juice Diet............................30

Three Ways to Avoid Cravings While Juice Fasting.....................30

Water Fasting to Lose Weight 31

Chapter 5: Ultimate Guide to Weight Solution........................ 33

Juicing to Manage Weight 33

Ten Brilliant Tips for Long-term Weight Loss........................35

Monitoring Weight Loss 37

Chapter 6: Choosing the Best Juicer 38

Juicer vs. Blender...39

Ten Different Types of Juicers.....................................40

Best Types of Juicers for Juice Fasting Purpose....................43

Chapter 7: Homemade Juicing for Weight Loss...................... 44

Homemade Juice is the Best 44

Making Juice without a Juicer 44

Storing Homemade Juice...45

Most Effective Storage Method 47

Chapter 8: Diet Plan for Weight Loss............................... 48

Vegetables Are Best For Shedding Pounds 48

Juices for Weight Loss 49

Eating and Drinking Enough...49

Going Off the Diet on a Bad Day 50

Having Red Meat during the Diet....................................51

Do I need a Formal Diet Program When I have Difficulty Losing
Weight? 51

Chapter 9: Juicing and Exercise for Weight Loss 52

How Much Should I Exercise for Weight Loss? 55

Chapter 10: Setting Your Goal for Weight Loss Solution 55

Being Realistic at Setting Goals 55

Compromises Made during the Diet and Being Prepared for them 56

Chapter 11: Ending Your Juice Fast Properly 58

A Simple Sequence to Break Your Juice Fast in One Week 59

Eating and Drinking Normally 60

Chapter 12: Juice Diet Recipes for Weight Loss 60

Chapter 1: Introduction

Juice fasting or having only freshly squeezed juices in your diet has become a popular way to reduce weight and tone up in recent years. Many celebrities like Olivia Wilde, Jessica Szohr and Nicole Richi among several others have been known to use juicing as an effective method to keep them fit and healthy. So why don't we follow their examples and discover the real benefits of juicing and find out how effective this can be for all of us who want to lose weight fast, remove the ugly bulge off our bellies and look slim like these celebrities?

'Juicing for Weight Loss' is a quick guide that carefully looks into every detail about what juicing is and how it can be used to achieve a significant weight loss. Reading through it, you will get to know about the benefits and other effects that juicing have for weight loss.

Worried about having put on too much weight? Don't be! That's because we will guide you step-by-step on how you can lose weight easily by treating yourself to tasty natural juices. We will be answering every question that you may have in your mind and clear all your doubts about juicing very shortly. So are you ready to begin losing weight by going on a journey of juicing?

What is Juicing?

Juicing means to extract the juices of fruits or/and vegetables by either squeezing them by hand or using a machine called 'juicer'. It brings out a colored and flavored watery content from the fruits or vegetables, both factors depending on what type of fruits or vegetables you use. For example, if you juice raw spinach, you are likely to get a green juice out of it with a slightly strong flavor.

Why Do the Juice Diet?

Juices are full of vitamins, minerals and antioxidants. All these are really good for you and your health. Antioxidants detoxify the bad toxins that your body creates all the time. As juices are water-based they fill you up quickly without having to eat much. They are low in calories with all the nutrients packed in a raw, easy-to-digest liquid form. So what happens is that you tend to take in fewer calories that automatically help to lose weight in a very short period of time. Homemade juices made from fresh fruits and vegetables are pure, natural and free from any additives, artificial colors or preservatives. That is why they are so healthy and good for you!

Understanding Juice Fasting

● What is it?

Juice fasting is a method of abstaining from food and having a juice diet instead. You make fresh home-made juices and do not buy the commercially available ones during the diet. These are consumed at regular intervals throughout the day for a certain period of time. It is a part of 'detox diet' (we'll explain very shortly what this means) that not only helps lose weight, but cleanses your body thoroughly

- What should and should not be consumed on a Juice Fast?

  Now while you're 'juice fasting', you should restrict yourself to juices extracted from organic fruits and vegetables and abstain from having calorie rich foods such as meat (whether red or white) eggs and dairy products. Other things you should avoid consuming include sugar, fizzy or alcoholic drinks, caffeine and wheat. What is recommended by experts is that you do not only avoid having these during your fast, but at least seven days before the detox diet begins. The diet should consist mainly of organic fruits, vegetables and beans.

The number of days the fast can last for varies from the person to person. A general recommendation is that you should consume between 32oz to 64oz of juice on a daily basis until the end of your fast However, the more you consume, the better it is. Any fruits and vegetables you like can be used. There are a few common ones that are particularly used during juicing. Typically, spinach, celery, carrot, kale, beans and other greens are used as vegetables. Among fruits, apples, pineapples, grapefruits, grapes, watermelons and cranberries are the most popular ones. You should also include plain water at room temperature and optionally herbal teas (without any sugar) in your diet.

Understanding Detox Diet

Earlier we said 'juice fasting' is a part of detox diet. But what is a detox diet?

Your body is constantly generating toxins that are bad for your health. You need to get rid of these toxic substances to maintain a healthy lifestyle. Your body's excretion system is meant to do this for you. So when you urinate, perspire or have a bowel movement, you're getting rid of these harmful substances present in your body. By detoxification, we try to make this system of removing harmful substances from our bodies more efficient. One way to do it is by going on a detox diet where you eat only those types of foods which are rich in antioxidants. You can achieve this target by juicing also. That's right! Juice detox helps to cleanse your body thoroughly, yet gently. Juices are full of substances called 'antioxidants'. Fresh juices also encourage the healing system of your body to work more efficiently and effectively. Hence, they make you feel fresh and revitalized. Juices are very light on your digestive system as they contain nutrients and minerals that are easily absorbed by your digestive system. This contributes to giving you more energy, clearer skin, and fewer digestive and other health issues.

Effective Weight Loss through Juicing

Juicing for weight loss can be not only effective, but very interesting to do and at the same time tasty as well. There is nothing like having fresh home-made juices using all your favorite fruits and vegetables. It is in fact one of the easiest and tastiest way to cut down on the excess fat accumulated in your body.

Although there is still no scientific evidence of it working well, many people have successfully and effectively lost weight by going on a juice fast. How does that work then? The answer is simple: Because most vegetables contain almost no fat and at the same time low in calories, you can easily cut down on calorie intake by being on a juice fast. You get all the nutrients present in the juice that your body can absorb and digest easily to keep you fit and healthy.

If you want to lose weight, you will have to cut down on your calorie intake. It's as simple as that. Since juices are low in calories and high in nutrients, it becomes easier to lose weight. Now if the RDA is 2000 calories for you and you take in, let's say, 1800 calories daily, you won't be giving yourself enough energy to carry on your day-to-day activities.

Hence, nature uses a clever system to help you survive by burning off the fat stored within your body to compensate for the loss, which is 200 calories in this case.

So by squeezing juices from the fruits and vegetables and drinking them daily without having the normal food, you provide your body with all the essential nutrients it needs, but no extra sugar or fat. Hence losing weight becomes easy and simple.

Let us assume you take in about 10 glasses of juice daily. If each one has 150 calories, you give yourself 1500 calories a day. This means 500 extra calories that your body still needs will be provided to you naturally when the excess fat in your body is burn. At this rate you should manage to shed off at least 1lb per week and in just three months' time, you can lose more than 12lbs! Amazing isn't it?

Goodbye Vitamins and Supplements!

That's right! Say good-bye to vitamins and supplements! You really don't need to take any supplements at all. What you're aiming to do is lose weight and cleanse your body by removing the harmful toxic substances present within it. Fruits and vegetables are rich in vitamins and minerals. Just to give you a fair idea an apple contains minerals like iron, potassium, phosphorous, magnesium, sodium, copper, zinc, manganese, calcium and traces of others minerals as well! It is also rich in vitamins such as Vitamin A, B1, B2, B6, C, E, Niacin, Folate, Pantothenic Acid and traces of a few other vitamins too. So imagine how many vitamins and minerals you obtain naturally if you use a combination of 3-4 different types of fruits and vegetables in your juice! So you essentially fulfill your body's requirements for vitamins and minerals by consuming the lovely, fresh, homemade juices you make using organic fruits and vegetables.

How Long Does It Take To Lose Weight On a Juice Diet?

Well, there is no definite answer to this unfortunately. It again varies from person to person. It depends on how much you have gained already, how much you look forward to losing, how devoted and determined you are to achieve this target, your genetics and most importantly how high is your metabolism (the capability of your body to burn food to release energy).

As with any other diet and exercise regimen you follow, you will not see results in just a couple of days' time. It may take several weeks before you start showing off results. You will need to be determined and it will work. You may feel dizzy and tired during the first few days and may want to give up, but this is normal. You need to have patience and determination to see actual results. It may take time, but it definitely works if you want to make it work. Some people take longer than others and some people just wouldn't be ready to follow the exact diet plan or even continue after some time.

Chapter 2: Nutritional Benefits of Juicing

We have already established the fact that juicing helps reduce weight and at the same time is very good for your health too. You will be absolutely amazed to find out how beneficial juices are for you. It is nutritious, helps with your metabolism, contains micro-nutrients that help in weight loss, flushes away toxic substances present in our bodies and fights diseases such as cancer. That's right! Juicing does help prevent cancer!

The advantages associated with juicing are endless.

Benefits of Juicing

Juicing is such a good idea for weight loss. Here are some of the reasons why you should consider it to lose weight:

1. It's Fun
Yes, it is so much fun to choose your favorite fruits and vegetables and squeeze them through the juicer to prepare your rich and healthy juice.

2. It's Easy
In all other diets, you have to follow a proper diet and exercise regimen. However, with juicing, all you need to do is choose your favorite juice recipes or create some of your own and literally let the juicer do the job for you. All you have to do is enjoy the delicious drink. And, without any doubt it is much easier to drink a glass of juice filled with nutrients than chew down a plate of food with the same amount of nutrients.

3. It's Yummy
Juices can be such a delicious treat to have. You can choose the fruits and vegetable you like to prepare for your very own juice.

4. There's so Much Variety
The best thing with juices is that you can try so many different fruits and vegetables and come up with a new combination and taste every time. If you have just four fruits and vegetables, you can create 10 different combinations with them easily. So imagine how many different ones would you be able to make if you have more?

5. Provides Vitamins and Minerals
Fruits and vegetables are full of vitamins and minerals. This means being on a juice diet provides you with all the essential nutrients your body needs to stay healthy. Say 'bye-bye' to vitamins and supplements as you no longer need them. You fulfill your requirements from natural sources! What could be better than that?

6. Brings Down Cholesterol Level

All the fried food and stuff rich in fat content increases the level of cholesterol in your body. Too much of it can block arteries and veins and cause heart problems. You do not only control your intake of cholesterol, but reduce the amount of bad cholesterol present within your body by having raw fruits and vegetables or their juices.

7. Helps Lose Weight Effectively

We have already established this fact and learned before how juicing works to help reduce weight. It is a fast, effective and easy method to cut down the excess fat accumulated in your body.

8. Detoxifies

Toxic substances are produced within your body all the time. If they are not eliminated properly, you could get one or more of the following problems:

- Your organs may start malfunctioning
- Muscles may become weak and body might start aching
- Brain functions may slow down
- Skin problems may arise and
- Your face might start looking dull and lifeless

Sounds dreadful, doesn't it? Worry not! Juicing is a solution to all these problems. The raw fruits and vegetables are rich in fiber which aids digestion and the antioxidants in them help detoxify and bring a natural glow to your face, hair, nails and skin.

9. Eliminates Acne Problems

The essential nutrients, vitamins, fiber and antioxidants present in the juices of raw fruits and vegetables effectively remove toxins from your body which are leading causes of acne. If you go on a juice diet, you'll notice in a few days' time how quickly your acne starts disappearing and you'll notice soon that your face gets a nice, fresh and healthy look.

10. Aids Digestion

The processed, cooked food we consume nowadays are full of fat, spices and artificial additives which require our digestive systems to work harder in order to break them down into useful substances that will release energy to our bodies. On the other hand, juices are in raw, unprocessed liquid forms that contain enzymes and make food very easy to digest. Wave good-bye to problems like gas, acidity, heartburn, acid reflux and other digestion problems simply by going on a juice diet!

11. Increases Immunity
Juices provide nutrients that help build immunity making you healthier and helping your body fight any harmful bacteria that may cause diseases.

12. It Has Anti-aging Properties
Did you know that juices contain all those ingredients that are used in the making of anti aging products? Yes that's true! Fruits and vegetables are naturally rich in nutrients that slow down the aging process and make you look young, fresh and youthful. Why spend a fortune on useless anti aging beauty products then?

We have just discussed twelve general benefits associated with juicing. There are countless others such as preventing diseases and making your organs work more efficiently, etc.

Four Benefits of Juicing Raw Fruits

Fruits are yummy and their juices are a treat to have. But what are the nutritional benefits of having juices and why is it important that we combine both the fruits and vegetables in our juices?

1.   Rich in Vitamins and Other Nutrients

Fruits are packed in vitamins, minerals and antioxidants for example all citrus fruits contain ascorbic acid (Vitamin C) which is very important for a healthy skin, helps prevent scurvy or bleeding gums and helps in the absorption of iron in our bodies. Some fruits such as apples, blackberries, gooseberries, grapes, prunes and citrus fruits are high in pectin, known to have health benefits such as lowering cholesterol and regulating the digestive tract.

2. Provide Instant Energy
Fruit juices contain sugars that are very quickly absorbed by our bodies in order to provide instant energy. Should you need to boost your energy levels, a glass of freshly squeezed fruit juice should do the job for you.

3. Rich in Minerals
Fruits contain minerals in quantities that you can't virtually get from any other raw sources of food. For instance avocados, guavas and bananas are rich in potassium and apples, pears, dates and raisins are all good sources of iron.

4. Pleasant Tasting
Fruit juices are sweet, pleasant to taste and have such lovely colors which appeal in every way to our senses. We can't resist sipping fruit juices. If you were to have vegetable juices all by themselves, you probably wouldn't have them as they don't taste, look and smell as good as the fruit juices do. Combining the two can bring better flavor and texture to the juice which would be more pleasant and easier to sip down.

Four Benefits of Juicing Raw Vegetables

We all love fruit juices, don't we? They taste good, smell good and have colors that are so pleasing to the eye. Then, why not just have fruit juices when on a juice diet? Well, vegetables have their own benefits which fruits cannot provide. Here are a few:

1. Low Sugar Content

Vegetables are lower in sugar content than fruits. If you consume fruit juices alone, you consume more sugar and hence more calories than if you combine the two together.

2. Helps Balance pH

Vegetables help in removing acidic waste from the body. This helps in balancing the overall pH of the body as well as the metabolism.

3. Essential Nutrients

Vegetables compensate for the essential nutrients that fruits are missing upon. They also include certain antioxidants, vitamins and folic acid, all of which are essential for your body. These essential nutrients help prevent diseases and boost immunity.

4. More Soluble Fiber

Vegetables contain a good amount of soluble fiber which helps absorb excess water from the colon and hence the feces are soft and watery making them easier to be excreted out, thereby getting rid of the harmful toxins, cholesterol and bad bacteria that can cause infections and diseases.

Preventing Diseases through Juicing

Juicing is not just meant for weight loss; it also helps prevent diseases. Diseases as serious as cancer!

Because juices help in detoxification, they can help in preventing diseases that can be caused by the presence of toxins and bad bacteria in our body. This naturally means all skins disease and infections. Acne breakouts can be prevented through the intake of raw juices.

Also diseases associated with digestion and organs of the digestive systems are also resolved through juicing. Those suffering from gastric problems, acidity or inflammation of stomach or intestines can use juicing to help them out. The cleansing action of raw juices helps prevent diseases and problems associated with the whole digestive and excretory system including, stomach, kidneys, liver, gall bladder, intestines and colon.

The colon present inside our bodies stores waste that is meant to be excreted out. If it stays there too long and is not removed, it can cause 'colon infections'. To cleanse the colon, juicing is a very effective method. Being on a liquid diet makes your stools easy to pass and along with them you get rid of all sorts of toxic substances and waste products that do your bodies no good.

Likewise, the largest organ present within our bodies that is the liver converts food into useful substance that is needed by our bodies. It produces enzymes that help digest food and together helps neutralize harmful toxins and wastes. Thus, the liver has very important functions to perform, but it always remains at great risk of contamination from toxins. To cleanse it and keep it functioning effectively raw fruit and vegetable juices act life savers.

You could improve your vision by consuming carrot juice, which is rich in Vitamin A or prevent scurvy by having orange juice that is rich in vitamin C or if you're anemic, fruits like apples that are rich in iron can compensate for your iron deficiency. In short the consumption of juices does actually help prevent countless diseases in a natural and effective way. If you make natural homemade juices a part of your healthy diet, you would not need to see a doctor again.

Micronutrients in Fruits and Vegetables That Enhance Weight Loss

Micronutrients are those nutrients that are present only in trace amounts in our food. Despite their small quantities, they are very important for our general health and well-being. These are required by our bodies to perform their functions efficiently and effectively. So in case you're trying to lose weight, the inclusion of micronutrients in your diet will help you lose those extra pounds in a more effective way. Luckily, fruits and vegetables contain the necessary micronutrients that your body needs to lose weight effectively. Here are a few examples of these along with their sources:

• Chromium

Chromium is found in small traces in certain fruits and vegetables such as tomatoes, onions and potatoes. It is one of the most crucial element that help shed the extra fat cells from our bodies. It does so by increasing the level of good cholesterol and improving the resistance to insulin in our bodies. If the body is deficient in chromium, the blood sugar levels rise automatically and you naturally begin to crave for sweet, high calorie food stuff.

• Alpha Lipoic Acid (ALA)

Alpha lipoic acid (ALA) increases the metabolic rate which means it helps convert food quickly into energy. The people you see around consuming so much food and yet remaining so slim and smart tend to have a high metabolic rate. Broccoli, spinach and chard are some sources of ALA. So make sure you include these in your diet the next time.

• Carnitine and Acetyl-L-carnitine

Carnitine acts in the presence of Omega -3 to increase our metabolic rate making it easier to lose weight whereas its derivative acetyl-L-carnitine helps transport the fatty acids to our cells so that they can be burned to release energy. These are found in meat, poultry and dairy products. Plant sources of these are avocados and asparagus.

Glutamine, DMAE, Gamma linolenic acid (GLA), DMAE (dimethylaminoethanol), Conjugated linoleic acid (CLA), Coenzyme Q10 (ubiquinone) are a few other micronutrients that aid weight loss in various different ways. These can all be found in trace quantities in juices made of fresh fruits and vegetables.

Five Major Advantages of Juicing Over Eating Whole Fruits and Vegetables

Now we all know that raw fruits and vegetables contain nutrients, micronutrients, antioxidants, vitamins, minerals and enzymes which have so many nutritional benefits. But why is there a need to juice them up? Why not just eat them raw and not juice them? Well the answer to these questions is that juicing is far more beneficial than having them whole. Here, we have listed a few for you:

1. Juices Contain all Essential Nutrients
Juicing extracts all the essential juices and nutrients present in fruits and vegetables.

2. Easy to Sip
Juices are easier to sip down than having to chew the whole fruits or vegetables.
3. Easy to Digest
Being in a liquid form and containing all the useful enzymes, they are easier to digest than whole fruits and vegetables.

4. More Nutritious
If equal quantities of both are consumed, juices would provide more nutrition than whole fruits and vegetables. That's because the indigestible fiber has been through juicing.

5. Taste Variations
Sometimes you just do not like the taste of certain fruits and/or vegetables. By juicing fruits and vegetables together, you tend to vary their taste and it becomes a lot easier to consume them in the form of juices rather than having them whole.

Chapter 3: The Side Effects of Juicing

Okay, so we know the benefits of juicing. It all sounds really good and safe to do. Then, what about the side-effects of juicing? Is there anything that is 'bad' associated with juicing? Unfortunately the answer is 'yes'. Like all things have their advantages and disadvantages, pros and cons, juicing is no exception. But relax, most of these symptoms are either temporary or non-serious and can be controlled if you do carry out your diet in the right way.

We'll discuss all possible symptoms of juicing and provide the answers to all the above questions related with those symptoms. This awareness will make your juicing diet more comfortable and easy to carry on. However, if you do not know what's happening and why, there are chances you may get confused and might even want to quit at some stage. So let's begin finding out the symptoms related to juicing:

1. Headaches
Some people might experience headaches for the first few days while on a juice diet. This is natural and there's nothing to worry. It comes because people may be addicted to caffeinated drinks like tea, coffee and coke. Giving them all up all of a sudden is not accepted by our bodies immediately and headaches show up as a consequence. They normally last 2-4 days and can be completely avoided by giving up on all forms of caffeine a week or two before the fast begins.

2. Food Cravings
Of course this can happen quite a lot of times in people who are on any sort of diet. The obvious reason for this is that it is human nature to tend to do things you are prohibited to do. So if on a diet you're asked to refrain from having fat-rich junk food stuff like pizzas, chips and burgers, you are likely to crave for all of these during the diet. If you successfully hold on to your cravings, they tend to go away in a few days' time.

3. Boredom

Sometime because you don't get to eat the things you want, you start getting bored very quickly. You might have noticed in your daily life that whenever you feel bored, chewing a chewing gum or having something sweet or biting on to biscuits or crunchy crisps really helps. Now imagine when you can't get to have any of these things, you naturally become overwhelmed by the feeling of ennui.

4. Anger and Frustration
At times you might feel very angry and frustrated just because you have been asked to refrain from foods and drinks that you really love. Don't worry if you become irritated easily during the diet! That's quite normal to happen.

5. Light Diarrhea
This is again something that would happen while on a juice diet. Nothing to worry about as this helps you get rid of all the toxic substances present within your body and give your body a thorough cleanse from inside.

6. Tiredness and Fatigue
It can occur because the detoxification process uses up most of the energy that normally keeps you active. This is again temporary and goes away in a couple of days.

7. Burning Sensation in the Anus
This is a very rare condition, but if it happens, there is no need to be worried about it. It is a sign that you are excreting out the toxic substances from your body. These toxins are acidic in nature and give you the hot or burning sensation during a bowel movement. You tend to feel much more relaxed immediately after the bowel movement as your body is free from toxins.

8. Nausea and Vomiting
Very few people experience this condition and it only lasts for about a day or two. It is caused by hunger pangs during the first few days and can be relieved by having lemon juice or drinks containing a bit of ginger. However, if it lasts longer you may get dehydrated and should see a doctor straight away.

9. Muscle and Body Pains

Again a very small percentage of people experience such pains and they last only for a couple of days. They occur in people who have very high levels of toxins in their bodies. Some people may experience temporary arthritis as well during the fast. The pains are not very sharp or unbearable, but if they're quit the fast go and see your doctor straight away.

10. Breakthrough Bleeding in Women
Breakthrough bleeding occurs when you start bleeding in between your periods. Although there could be many causes of this, one such cause of breakthrough bleeding in women is rapid weight loss. It has nothing to do specifically with juicing, but it is related to weight loss and can very rarely occur if you're on a juicing diet and losing weight rapidly.

It is the sudden and abrupt change in your eating habits that can cause the unexpected bleeding to occur, but it only happens if you have lost too much weight over a very small span of time. This is hardly ever the case. However, if it does happen to you, there is no need to worry unless it happens more than once. You should consult a doctor to investigate the matter. Sometimes it is stressed related or a sudden change in your life could cause it too specially if you are on birth control pills.

11. Missing a Period
Although a missed period is generally regarded a sign of pregnancy or a consequence of breast feeding, this is not always the case. Periods can be missed due to a number of reasons and weight loss is one of them. Once again we'd emphasize the point that this doesn't in any way relate to the juicing diet. It is just an after effect of weight loss. It is very uncommon for this to happen, but if you tend to lose too much weight over a very short period of time, there are chances that you might miss your period. This is very normal so don't be over concerned about it. However, if you miss your periods for more than a month, it is worth doing a pregnancy test, stop dieting immediately and see your doctor as soon as possible.

12. Depression

Due to low-calorie intake when on a juice diet, the blood sugar level is likely to drop and this can lead to depression. Seeing other people enjoying normal food can sometimes make you feel depressed too during the first few days. But don't worry this is not a very serious problem and goes away with time.

13. Bad Breath and Body Odor
Bad breath and body odor due to excessive sweating are quite common symptoms of juicing and are signs of toxic wastes being eliminated from your bodies. Unfortunately not much can be done about it, except keeping yourself clean. Make sure you take a shower daily and brush twice a day at least to keep the bad smells at bay.

14. Parched Throat and Dry Lips
Very few people will experience a dry parched throat and feel thirsty time and again, despite taking in a lot of juices.

Again, this goes away in a few days and it shows that your body is eliminating all the harmful toxic substances that were trapped within it. Don't worry much about this and keep consuming as much liquid as you can. Just make sure you're not losing too much water else you will get dehydrated.

15. Swollen Ankles
Although not very common, some people might experience swollen ankle and puffy feet which may make them feel uncomfortable. It is perhaps due to the intake of too much liquid which starts accumulating around your feet if you're standing for too long. Keeping the feet elevated does bring comfort, but if it does not go away in a few days' time, consult your physician as it could be something more serious.

16. Sore Body
Your bodies tend to become a bit sore for a few days while on a juice fast. The reason behind is the consumption of a lot of liquid. This should generally go away in a 3-4 days but, if it doesn't, please make an appointment with your doctor to find out if everything is okay. Usually it is not a serious problem, but at times it can be and needs to be sorted out as soon as possible.

These are some of the most common symptoms of juicing and most of these will go away in a few days. If you experience any problems other than these, feel very weak or are not sure what's happening, it is best to go and speak to your doctor about it rather than wait for the problem to go away on its own.

Low Fiber, Protein and Fat Intake during a Juice Diet: Cons

Fiber is very important for your body. A drawback of juicing is that when the juice is extracted from the juicer, you leave the pulp of the fruits and vegetables behind. This is fiber.

The intake of fiber is necessary because it helps in bowel movements and in regulation of metabolism within our bodies. It also plays an important role in lowering cholesterol level.

Protein, again, is a very important constituent of a healthy diet. It can be found in meat, poultry, fish lentils and beans. It is responsible for the general growth of cells, muscles, tissues, hair and nails, building of antibodies and is a source of energy as well. Some fruits and vegetables contain no protein while others only have a small amount so by being on a juice diet, we're not actually are on a 'healthy' diet.

Fat is always considered bad for health, but the truth is our bodies do need a little amount of fat to maintain a healthy diet and an active lifestyle. Fat gives you the most amount of energy as compared to carbohydrates (sugars) and proteins. The excess of anything is bad and the same goes for fat because this is what starts accumulating in our bodies, making us 'fat' and causing heart and other health problems. Fruits and vegetables contain little or no fat at all. All sorts of nuts, dairy products, meat and eggs are good sources of fat.

So if you decide to go entirely on a juice fast, beware that besides all its benefits, you are also depriving yourself from essential nutrients such as proteins, fat and fiber. Make sure you do not continue doing your fast too long otherwise you might end up putting yourself in trouble.

Not Losing Weight When on a Juice Diet

Let's face it: juice diet has plenty of benefits and has worked wonders on some, but it may not just work for others because of their genetics or for several other reasons. Here, we will try to tell you about every possible reason which obstructs you from losing weight while on a juice diet. It is good to know whether the juice diet will work for you or not before starting on one to avoid disappointment later.

1. Genetics

Family history and genes play a vital role in weight loss. Some people actually have low metabolism rate and even if they eat very little, they just tend to put on weight.

2. Age

When you're young, the motivation to lose weight and your tendency to do it is really high. As you start getting older, you metabolism slows down and it becomes difficult, though not impossible, to lose weight quickly.

3. Lack of Motivation

Motivation is the key to success in any aspect of life. If you aren't motivated or determined to lose a pound or two a week, you won't change, no matter how hard you try. Your brain needs to know what you wish it to do and then once the target is set; it becomes easier to achieve the goal.

Having friends and family around who are doing the same or encouraging you to achieve your weight loss goal can help a great deal

4.   Negative Attitude

Some people just wouldn't try going on a diet saying; 'It isn't for me'. If you think so, then you're right, it's not for you. It is meant for optimistic people who think they can do it. Unless you remain positive and stay focused on what you want to do, you can't achieve anything, not even weight loss.

5.   Boredom

Boredom is a side-effect of juice fasting. When you get bored, you want to munch on something like crisps and on a juicing diet, you can't do that. If you can't keep control on yourself and are secretly munching on a packet of crisps every two to three days, you're just ruining everything. What weight loss you may achieve is gained through snacking!

6.   Improper Diet Plan

One reason because of which you might not be losing your weight could be because you're not following your juice diet plan accurately. You could be using too many fruits with high sugar content or having more than the recommended amounts of juices.

7.   You Can't Resist Cravings

Sometimes you may find that you can't hold on to your cravings so you start eating foods that you've been refrained from eating. Even if you treat yourself to a slice of pizza or a small packet of crisps every few days, you are gaining extra calories. There is simply no use of the juice diet if you do that because eating such stuff helps you gain weight faster than you lose it.

8.   Stress and Depression

Sugars from juice give you a burn away quickly releasing energy in an instant. However, that goes away and leaves you with too much insulin. This in turn throws off your serotonin cycle and causes you to be depressed. Therefore, depression comes naturally as a side-effect of juicing.

Stress and depression are both really bad for your health. If you feel stressed, you tend to consume more food than required without thinking about any harm they can do to you. Likewise, you tend to do a lot of comfort eating when you're depressed. Also, when you're stressed or/and depressed, your body releases a hormone, which is responsible for storing fat. So the more emotional problems you have, the more fat you tend to store making you gain weight rather than lose it. Hence, it is important you remain stress free throughout the diet plan and better still sort out your emotional problems before you start one.

9. Lack of Potassium, Micronutrients and Minerals

All these nutrients, as we've discussed before, help a great deal in weight loss. If you do not include enough fruits and vegetables which contain these essential nutrients and micronutrients, you'd simply fail to lose weight.

10. Sleeplessness

The lack of sleep is known to lead too many health problems including weight gain. Not getting enough rest interferes with the normal body mechanisms including metabolism. Just stay calm, relaxed and sleep for 6-8 hours daily to make your juicing diet plan or any other plan work for you.

Juicing is a very effective way to lose weight, but it may have side-effects. It is not necessary that you will be experiencing any of these, but awareness is important so that you know what to do if a problem occurs.

Chapter 4: Effective Fasting for Weight Loss

Having known all the advantages and disadvantages of a juicing diet, if you've still decided to use juicing as a method to lose weight, bravo! Yeah, we really mean it because you have the courage to take up the challenge no matter what. Well done! And, when you have this mind-set and determination to shed off the extra pounds, nothing can stop you from achieving this target.

You can achieve weight loss easily through a juice fast provided you do it in an effective manner. This chapter will focus on how you can use juice fasting as an effective method for weight loss.

Before You Begin

Are you ready to begin your juice fasting journey? Wow, you look pretty enthusiastic about it! Why wait, then? Let the journey begin! But wait! There are certain people who shouldn't be doing this fast. Check the list below to find out whether you're one of those or not:

- Women who are pregnant or breast-feeding or those who think they could be pregnant
- Those who're suffering from diseases of the kidney and liver and serious, chronic diseases such as ulcerative colitis, cancer, terminal illness, epilepsy
- People suffering from diabetes or even low blood sugar
- People who've had or about to have a surgery in the near future
- People suffering from malnutrition or those who're underweight or anemic
- People who are on certain medications.

It is always best to consult a doctor or a qualified nutritionist who can tell you whether or not you can start a juice diet.

Beginning the Fast: When and How?

To start your fast, it is a really good idea to have a smooth transition from having rich, heavy solid foods to liquid juices. You do not want to give your body a sudden shock. Do you?

Here are some useful tips to make this transition smooth:

•	It may sound like a good idea that you should start your fast in the winter months so that your body doesn't lose too much water and make you feel dehydrated, experts think spring is the most suitable time of the year to start the fast.

•	Cut down on your caffeine, alcohol and nicotine consumption before beginning the fast gradually that is if you drink three cups of tea a day, bring it down to two about 2-3 of weeks before the fast and then to just one and finally to nil a few days before you begin the fast.

•	You shouldn't be taking any aspirin or painkillers during the fast so make sure you can bear your head and body aches.

•	Consume cooked vegetables, salads, fruits, and juices a few weeks before fast begins. Avoid meat, dairy, poultry, fish or foods high in fat.

•	Limit your foods to raw salads, juices, fruits and vegetables.

•	As the fast approaches nearer, you could start cutting down more on solids and consuming more juices and liquids such as you could have only a glass of juice at breakfast, some salad and fresh fruits at lunch and again salad with a glass of juice for dinner.

• Try eating nothing but watery fruits and vegetables a couple of days before the fast begins. These may include melons, lettuce, citrus fruits and grapes.

Following these tips it becomes easier to move onto a diet full of juices and you're less likely to have any of the symptoms we mentioned in the previous chapter. If you fail to follow the simple rules or do not follow the diet plan as it is, you might end up getting dizzy, dull, and weak, depressed, bored and may end up gaining weight rather than losing it.

How Long Should a Juice Fast Last?

A juice fast typically lasts for three days and is required to occur intermittently, but this can vary from person to person depending on how much weight they are capable of losing and how much weight loss is actually required to be lost.

Sometimes a juice fast can be longer and may be required to be taken up for several weeks. It is important, however, that this be done under medical supervision and proper monitoring to ensure that nutrient deficiencies don't come as a consequence. That's primarily because long-term juice fasting can be detrimental as it deprives you of some very essential nutrients such as fiber, proteins and fat all of which are necessary to maintain a healthy way of life.

Top Ten Tips for Effective Fasting

Here are some useful tips that will help achieve better results in terms of weight loss and detoxification.

1. Consume between 32oz and 64oz of juices daily while on a juice fast.

2. Along with the juices, try to drink six to eight glasses of water.

3. Use only fresh organic fruits and vegetables to extract juices. In case they aren't available, wash the fresh fruits and vegetables thoroughly.

4. Drink the juices immediately after being squeezed. Do not consume left over juices as they can give rise to infections and diseases.

5. Consume the juices of as many fresh green leafy vegetables as you can as they're packed with goodness.

6. Avoid consuming juices made of fruits alone. Use a combination of both fruits and vegetables.

7. Discard the tops of root vegetables such as carrots and parsnips and seeds and stones from fruits such as prunes and peaches before extracting their juices.

8. Do not use the peel of citrus fruits or fruits with hard rough skins such as pineapples for juicing.

9. Avoid using fruits and vegetables like bananas, avocados or sweet corns as these have high calorie content in them.

10. If you're fasting for the first time and doing it alone, start with a day's fast and then after a few days you can fast for 3-5 days if necessary.

Eating Solids during a Juice Fast

A juice fast is strictly designed around drinking juices and water. Solids are not usually allowed. And, if the diet plan is followed accurately, it shouldn't make you feel weak and dizzy. However, some diet plans allow the consumption of one meal during the day while others allow having salads and fresh fruits, vegetables and nuts during the diet plan. Whatever the plan maybe, following it exactly will help you get the best results out of it. It is a good idea to get yourself monitored if you're fasting for more than 3-5 days so that your body doesn't lack in essential nutrients making you weak and feel sick.

Taking Antidepressants on a Juice Diet

Ideally you shouldn't go on a juice diet if you're prone to depression. If however, your doctor suggests you can, then there's no stopping you for sure. Continue taking antidepressants like you have been during the fast as well. Quitting them all of a sudden is not a good idea according to experts because they can have their own side-effects and can bring some serious problems too.

On the other hand, if depression comes to you as a symptom of fasting try not to take antidepressants in this case. Overcome your depression, but indulging yourself in other activities such as reading books, watching TV, talking to friends, doing gentle exercises or yoga or generally anything that makes you feel happy.

Three Ways to Avoid Cravings While Juice Fasting

It can be really hard to avoid cravings during any kind of fasts. They may develop as a consequence of the detoxification process. The problem is that if you have no control on these, you end up in a mess. The whole effort you put in starting and actually doing the fast is flushed down the drain. Besides, you tend to put on weight instead of losing it.

1. Distract Yourself

This is perhaps the easiest way, though not the best one to control your cravings. Just go out, watch a movie or a TV program that you like, call a friend or do anything that you like to and keeps you busy, except eating something, of course.

2. Avoid Sweeteners

Any type of juices you consume should be free from any sweetening agents, natural or artificial. If you use these, you are more likely to crave for sweet things. Consume fresh juices without any additives to fill you up.

3. Use relaxation Techniques

Sometimes doing gentle exercises, going out for a walk, yoga, and meditation all can help you relax and think more about the benefits you will be able to reap after you've finished doing your fast instead of the present cravings or other side-effects you might experience.

Water Fasting to Lose Weight

Like juice-fasting, water fasting can be another good method to lose weight effectively. You could use a combination of juice and water fasting or merely water fasting on its own to achieve a significant weight loss. Let us find out what water fasting is and how can it be used to achieve weight loss.

•   The Importance of Water in Our Lives

Three fourths of the earth is covered in water and our bodies too are made up of 50%-60% of water. It plays a vital role in making our blood more 'watery', so that it can easily flow around the bodies, transporting oxygen, nutrients to where they are needed.

Although you do get a lot of water from your homemade juices, it is also important that you drink about six to eight glasses of water during your juice fast.   Water will help in the detoxification process by flushing out the toxic wastes out of our bodies.   It will also act as an appetite suppressant that will make you feel full without needing to eat anything.   During your juice diet, if you feel hungry or crave for food just go and get a glass of water to fill you up.

You will then naturally tend to lose weight quickly and easily because water has virtually no calories at all!

•   Water Fasting: What, When, How and Why?
Like juice fasting, water fasting is another way to lose weight quickly. All you do while on water fast is keep yourself hydrated by drinking plenty of water and eat and drink nothing else. Of course you can lose a large amount of weight over a short period of time, but how much you lose again varies from one person to another. Some people would easily lose up to 4lbs per day, but that again depends on your metabolism.

Just as in the case of a juice fast, you can't water fast for a very long time because you do not get any nutrients to survive on. A day or at the most a couple of days should be good enough. Before the beginning of the water fast you need to change your eating, and drinking habits just like you do in the case of a juice fast. You should bring down your appetite and consume only juices and water a couple of days before you start so that you do not give your body a sudden shock.

Once you start, just consume water for a day or two and see how drastically you lose your weight. Doing so every few weeks or so will bring shocking results in a very short time that you will be amazed to see. However, it is important you consult a dietician, nutritionist or a doctor before you start. There are certain people with certain medical conditions or undertaking certain medications who aren't supposed to go on water fast.

•   Side Effects of Water Fasting and How to Overcome Them
Water fasting can be effective, but has certain side-effects. The most common ones are dizziness and blackouts. Avoid working too much and get plenty of rest to avoid getting dizzy or feeling too weak. However, if you experience any other symptoms, it is best to quit fasting and get an expert's advice.

Chapter 5: Ultimate Guide to Weight Solution

We have discovered by now juicing is one effective way to lose weight. We have also looked into the best ways we can use it to make the most out of it, but we are also aware you still have several questions and doubts about this plan. Don't worry, as we promised earlier, we are going to clear all your doubts and answer all your questions throughout this report so that before you start, you know exactly what is the best for you and what should you be doing in case you have   problems.

This chapter will guide you, as the name suggests already, to the solutions to weight loss and how juicing can be used to manage weight loss.

Juicing to Manage Weight

Juicing is an optimal solution to lose weight that comes with countless other health benefits. But can it be used to manage weight? Of course it can be! It is, however, not cast with a magical spell so do not expect a colorful glass of juice to just burn away the extra fat cells. You will unfortunately still need to keep yourself active and fit through some sort of exercise or even a walk to increase your metabolism.

Gaining too much? Simply go on a juice diet for a few days and when you have achieved the optimal weight loss, just go off the diet and come back to your normal lifestyle.

But what if you have lost too much weight? This is when you need to be careful. Find out the root cause of the problem. If you have lost weight all of a sudden without you trying to do it, see a doctor at once to find out what is wrong. It could be related to hormonal imbalance, stress or a thousand other reasons. Some may not be too serious, but others can be.

Having known the problem, you can adjust your diet accordingly. At this time, you can eat healthy food and drink juices as a part of a healthy diet, but do not be completely dependent on them as you would in a juice fast. Having done this, you can carry on with your normal lifestyle and routine until you have gained enough according to your gender, height and weight. These factors play an important role in calculating your BMI (body mass index) which tells you exactly whether you are underweight, overweight or normal. You can find BMI calculators online which are very easy to use when you Google search for them.

What you need to do to manage weight loss is to commit to make juicing a part of your lifestyle. Soon you will discover its benefits making way to you. Being creative with juicing and coming up with new ideas and recipes all of which you can modify according to your taste and needs cannot just be beneficial for you, but fun too.

If you do not fancy going on a juice fast, simply have a glass of freshly squeezed juice using a combination of fresh fruits and vegetables and sip it before each meal. You will notice how quickly you fill yourself up.

You will be eating fewer calories and drinking more nutrient-rich juices, helping you keep good control over your weight and benefitting from goodness nature has packed in the fresh produce at the same time.

Ten Brilliant Tips for Long-term Weight Loss

Sure you can drastically lose weight through juicing or some other form of diet, but to maintain this weight loss, here are a few tips so that you remain fit and active for the rest of your lives:

1. Count Your Calories
For an average person, the RDA is 2000 calories. If you count the number of calories, you consume daily, you can keep track of how much you've eaten and whether you need more or not. Almost all packaged food that is available today does have a nutrition chart on the packaging. Follow what amounts you consume and how many calories it totals too. It should be more or less around 2000 calories during the entire day, no matter what you eat. This is assuming that you are only trying to maintain your weight and not losing it. If you are trying to lose weight, your calorie intake should be less than 2000 daily.

Please note that the RDA can vary from a person to a person. It can be higher than 2000 calories for men who are tall and broad and lower for women who are short and slim. Speak to a nutritionist, fitness expert or dietitian to help you find out how many calories you need daily, if you are unsure.

2. Consume Healthy Foods
Try choosing healthier options for foods over junk ones. Consume more fruits and vegetables either lightly cooked or raw. Eat plenty of salads and fresh produce. Avoid unhealthy, junk and processed foods such as chips, burgers and pizzas. It's okay to have them once or twice a year, but not every other day as they have a very high-calorie count and can let you gain weight far quicker than you can imagine.

3. Have Control Over Your Cravings
You might not want to gain weight, but you easily can if you cannot control your cravings. You have to learn to distract yourself or participate in activities that will make you forget about these carvings.

4. Set Goals

Have a diary where you can write down certain rules you need to follow and targets you want to achieve. For instance, you can plan to consume only one form of starch daily; it will be bread, pasta, rice or potatoes or have at least one meal, which is just a salad and nothing else or consume one glass of skimmed milk at night.

Whatever you plan, just write it down in your diary or a piece of paper and attach it to your fridge so that you see it and follow it. It works for many people when they have it written, and they can see it every now and then to remind themselves of it rather than having it all in their heads.

5. Have Patience
Be patient with everything you do. Don't expect you will fast one day and lose your weight the next day. Our bodies don't work this way. They take time to accept changes and manipulate them. So don't give up and carry on with your goals patiently.

6. Get Some Motivation
We've stressed on being motivated to carry on your diet plan every now and then. Trust us, it really helps. If you live all by yourself, and you have to do something, you probably won't because of the lack of motivation. However, with the support of friends and family, things become a lot easier to do.

If you're eating healthy and others in your family are not, you can be de-motivated easily. Encourage them to consume healthy foods like yourself by explaining the benefits of healthy foods and the drawbacks of eating calorie-rich food. If you all work as a team, it can be very easy to lose weight in the long-term too.

7. Exercise
It's not all about eating. You have to keep yourself active and fit. Exercising to keep your metabolism high, makes you sweat and burn off those extra fat cells. So
Plan a workout. It doesn't have to be tough and hard work. You could plan to walk at a good fast pace for one hour each day if you can't run or jog.

8. Change your Life Style

Change your lifestyle a bit. If you go to the shopping center by car, which is just 20 minutes away from your house, consider walking there or ride your bicycle. If you can't walk up to there, just park your car further away from the entrance. That way, you will have to walk a bit to the entrance and come back with bags the same distance by walking, giving you a bit of work out.

In your house even, you can work harder at cleaning, gardening or washing up. For example, if you wash all your clothes in the washing machine and take them away in a basket outside all at once, try to take a few at a time and hang them dry on the washing line, come back for more, hang them again and continue doing so until you're done with them all.

9. Cut Down on Fizzy Drinks and Alcohol
Cut down on your sugar intake not just by eating less dessert and sweet things, but by avoiding fizzy drinks and alcohol. Both of these are very high in sugar and can instantly build up on calories. If you need something to drink, why not just drink a healthy homemade juice or even fresh water? The more you drink these, the more quickly you will fill-up, and the less will be your intake of calories.

10. Get Good Sleep
Those who can't get a good sleep at night are more prone to gain weight. So to maintain an active and healthy lifestyle, make sure you get enough sleep. Usually six to eight hours of sleep is recommended for a healthy person. Are you getting enough?

Monitoring Weight Loss

As we mentioned earlier some people will not lose weight as easily as compared to others unfortunately because of a low metabolism rate or their family history or negative attitude. Whether you are losing weight or not that has to be monitored closely.

Don't just buy weighing scales for yourself and check your weight every day and get disappointed. It doesn't work that way. There's a proper way to check weight. Firstly, don't do it on a daily basis. Do it every week or every five days. Set a day, a time and check your weight by wearing minimal or no clothes on the same day and same time of the day. It is only then you will figure out whether you're losing weight or not, and how much weight you have lost.

It takes time for your body to show a change so be patient with yourself.

Usually experts recommend having your weight checked early in the morning before breakfast (that is before you eat or drink anything and without putting on any clothes). If you do the same the next week at the same time, you should be able to see some visible change. This change will keep you motivated to carry on with what you're doing. If you keep checking daily, you will see no change at all for several days, and you might give up easily. So please do not do that!

Don't let your emotions get into your way while you're on a diet. Weight loss isn't something easy and straightforward to achieve. You need determination, devotion, concentration, motivation, perseverance and the will to do it. If you feel good about what you're doing and what you've achieved, then you can continue easily no matter how tiny the weight loss may be. Encourage yourself and say 'Bravo! Good job! I have lost 2lbs now so 10lbs shouldn't be a problem; I can do it!'

Whether or not you lose your weight after a certain time, there's no need to worry at all. Just relax and let your body do its job while you give your best shot at controlling your weight.

Make an effort on your end and you can surely achieve anything you desire!

Chapter 6: Choosing the Best Juicer

Here we'll try to learn a bit more about a juicer, its functions, its types, which one suits your needs answer similar questions related to this machine.

Juicer vs. Blender

We are sure some of you might be thinking about using a blender instead for juicing or maybe worried about the differences between the two.

Blenders will blend together everything you add in it whereas juicers tend to extract the juices of fruits and vegetables and remove the pulp of these. This means using a blender will result in a thicker more nutritious juice as it contains all the fiber as well whereas a juicer will bring out a more watery juice. Despite lacking fiber in them, juices have numerous advantages over the blended smoothies that we've learnt about earlier.

Blenders can be used to make delicious smoothies, but for a juice diet, it is preferred to use a proper juicer to prepare your juices. Now a blender being off the list, the next question that arises is 'What is the best type of juicer?'

Juicers are available in a number of different types. All these extract juices but function differently. We need to look into each type and understand how it functions before deciding the best one for our needs. Some important considerations to have in mind before buying one are listed below:

1. Budget
You might have a budget in mind and may want to spend accordingly. Some juicers are cheap while others are way too expensive. If a juicer satisfies most of your needs within your budget, why go for an expensive option.

2. Ease of Use

Juicers vary on the basis of how you can operate them to make your juice. Some juicers will provide you with fresh juice in a matter of seconds and all at once.

However, they may be hard to clean when removing the pulp. Others will take time to juice, but remove the pulp while juicing, making them very easy to clean.

3.   What can be juiced?

This is one of the most important considerations. Not all juicers will juice everything you want. Some are dedicated to juice only certain fruits and vegetables. You need to check whether the juicer you're buying can juice all the fruits and vegetables that you intend to juice.

4.   Efficiency

You must check the efficiency of a juicer. Juicers do not tend to remove all the juice. Ask your retailer about what percentage of juice does the juicer you wish to go for extract or how much is wasted with the pulp. Cheap juicers will waste a lot of juice. This means that if you can make a glass of apple juice with five apples normally, you might need 6-8 apples for a cheap juicer to make a glass of juice. In the long-term this may turn out to be very expensive for you. So judge carefully whether it's better to invest on a good juicer or not.

5.   Warranty

Like all electrical appliances, juicers also come with a warranty. Check for how long it is covered because anything can go wrong with electrical and electronic appliances and in case something does within a year or three years may be; you can get a replacement or repair for free from the manufacturer.

Now there is no such thing as a best juicer. Each one has its own pros and cons. As we look into the types of juicers, we'll also have a sneak peek at their advantages and disadvantages.

Ten Different Types of Juicers

1. Centrifugal Spinning Juicers

In such types of juicers, the fruits and vegetables are fed through the feed chute on top of the machine. A flat spinning blade rotates around at 3600 rpm to shred the produce and juice is extracted by the spinner.

The pulp comes out dry, and all the juice can be collected in a container. However, a centrifuge spinning juicer cannot be used to collect all the juice at once. It has to be stopped as soon as it fills up with pulp. The pulp has then got to be removed before you proceed with the rest of the juicing. Another disadvantage of this juicer is that although it can juice, a variety of produce, leafy greens, barley grass, sprouts or wheat-grass is an exception.

2. Centrifugal Pulp Ejectors

These juicers work exactly in the same manner as Centrifugal Spinning Juicers. However, they allow continuous operation as the pulp is continuously removed out of the machine as the juicer is operated. This pulp can be collected in a separate wastebasket. Hence, they are easier to clean as well. These juicers spin at about 6,300 rpms, but are a bit nosier.

Like Centrifugal Spinning Juicers, These juicers are not good for juicing leafy greens, barley grass, sprouts or wheat-grass.

3. Commercial Centrifugal Juicers

Such juicers are the same as Centrifugal Pulp Ejectors. The only difference is that these are meant for commercial juice. They can juice very large quantities and are made up of heavy-duty parts to withstand the pressure of juicing into a commercial environment.

4. Single Auger Masticating Juicers

These are perhaps the best ones available for juicing in the sense that they are:

• 	very quiet,

- do not oxidize the juice,
- run at a very low rpm and
- Are great for juicing leafy green veggies, barley grass, wheat grass which centrifugal machines fail to juice.

The only disadvantages perhaps would be that juicing takes a bit of time as the motor runs slowly and that the fruits and vegetables need to be cut into small pieces as the feed chute is a bit small. Soft fruits such as grapes should be juiced with other hard fruits adding each one after the other to avoid backing up the machine.

5.   Dual Stage Single Augers

This works in the same manner as a single auger, but is more efficient because of the availability of a dual stage screen. This helps extract more juice in less time. The pulp comes of drier, and the juice isn't too foamy.

6.   Vertical Single Auger Juicers

These are upright juicers similar to single auger masticating ones except that they are upright and hence space-savers for storage in your kitchen. You get good-quality juice for any kind of fruit and veggies you add. The feed chutes are large so you don't need to chop or dice your produce. In fact, you can do juice fruits with pits and stones such as peaches and plums without having to remove them first.

7.   Twin Gear Press

These are one of the best kinds of juicers available because:

- they are very quiet,
- extract most of the juice leaving behind a very dry pulp,
- they rotate at a very low rpm,
- the juice is not oxidized or its quality is not deteriorated,
- Can juice all types of fruits and vegetables including leafy greens.

The only disadvantage of this is that while feeding the produce in the machine you need a bit of pressure to push it all in. For people suffering from arthritis, this machine is surely a no, no!

8. Masticating Juicers

These juicers function by crushing the fruits and vegetables first and then by squeezing them through a stainless steel screen. There is no need to dice the fruits and vegetables before feeding them in the chute. Often they come with extra attachments to allow multipurpose use and hence are very versatile.

9. Wheat-grass Juicers

These are single auger masticating types specifically designed to juice leafy greens, wheat-grass and barley grass. Of course, they can be used to juice all other fruits and vegetables as well. They can be either manual or electric.

10. Citrus Juicers

These juicers will only juice citrus fruits such as lemons, oranges and grapefruits. They are quiet and easy to clean as well.

Best Types of Juicers for Juice Fasting Purpose

Experts recommend the use of single or dual augers (horizontal or vertical) or masticating type ones or twin gear presses because they all can juice all types of produce, including the leafy greens and grass. You may find various models of these available in the market at different prices, and you can select the one that best meets your needs and budget.

Chapter 7: Homemade Juicing for Weight Loss

There are so many brands out there in the market selling juices at affordable prices, but throughout this report we have emphasized using fresh fruits and vegetables to produce your own juices in the comfort of your home. That's because homemade juices are simply the best.

Homemade Juice is the Best

Commercially available ones may be convenient and cheap, but most of them are made of concentrates or contain many additives and preservatives which we obviously want to avoid when we are trying to detoxify and lose weight at the same time. Furthermore, juices tend to lose their nutrients immediately (within seconds) after being squeezed so that it is best to consume them as soon as possible. The packaged ones cannot be in any way as good as the homemade ones for sure.

Okay so now having known how good homemade juice is we now have to make a determination now that we'll consume only fresh homemade juices made from organic produce (whenever possible) throughout the juice diet. That being said, we will of course need a juicer to extract our juice efficiently.

Making Juice without a Juicer

In the previous chapter, we already explained all the types of juicers available in the market and also highlighted the ones which are best for our juicing needs. However, a juicer can be an expensive buy. We understand that not everyone can afford to have one. So what? Should they refrain from going on a juice diet? Or what if your juicer breaks down while you're on a fast? Should you discontinue? The answer is 'No'. There should be some method of extracting the juice without one. Of course, there isn't one method, there are several. We'll explain how to do so in the easiest manner here.

Okay so all you need is a blender and a sieve.

Basically it is a three step process:

1. Preparation
Just prepare your fruits and vegetables which you wish to juice by cutting them and removing the pits, stones or seeds and stalks where necessary.

2. Blending
Put all the prepared produce in the blender along with some water and whizz until it's nice and smooth. You've got your smoothie ready!

3. Sieving
Now to get the juice out of it and remove the pulp, you have to sieve your smoothie. An ordinary sieve you use for straining pasta or rice has holes quite wide so it will allow some pulp through pass through it. It can be used if nothing is available, but ideally, you shouldn't be using them. The best type of sieve you can use is either a paint straining bag or a nut milk bag which could be purchased at DIY stores, Ebay, Amazon or several other online stores.
Citrus fruits can be juiced by hand directly and then sieved directly or the juice can be blended with other fruits and vegetables in a blender.

Storing Homemade Juice

Your juice is ready to drink straight away as soon as it is ready. But what if you make more juice than you require? Should you consume only what you need and discard the rest? Ideally you should drink your juices as soon as you can. They tend to oxidize and lose nutrients in no time and if left longer can be harmful for consumption.

To avoid wastage, always try to prepare quantities that you can consume immediately. However, there are times when you have a very busy routine and can't find time to make a glass of juice every time. In such cases, it is very handy to juice large quantities and store them away for use later. Here, we'll discuss some very easy ways to store homemade juices such that they are not harmful for later use.

First let's make it clear that you can't store all types of juices and those that you can be stored forever. How long a juice can be stored for depends on three factors namely:

1.   Juicing Method
What type of juicer you use plays a vital role in deciding the life of your juice. Some juicers like dual press or single augers run at a very low rpm meaning that there is a very little change in the temperature of juice, and they do not oxidize too quickly. The quality of such juices is simply great and they last longer.

2.   Produce Used
Fruit juices made from apples or pears, and vegetable juices made using leafy greens tend to oxidize very quickly. On the other hand, citrus fruits contain ingredients, which delay the oxidation process and these usually last very long.

3.   Storage Method
How you store your juice also decides the life of the juices. Certain types of air tight storage containers allow juices to be kept much longer than any other ones.

4.   Temperature
As with any other perishable item, juices stored in a fridge or freezer will last much longer than if they are stored at room temperature. So you need to be careful to store them in a cool dry place. In that way, bacteria cannot germinate quickly enough to spoil the whole juice.

Most Effective Storage Method

Okay now we know the factors that can degrade or deteriorate since the quality of the juice, so we need to incorporate all the tips above to make an effective storage method.

1. Pour your juice straight away into airtight glass containers or bottles. Research shows glass containers are better for storage than plastic ones as they do not tend to react with the juice at all. If you sterilize these first and chill those in the fridge a few hours before you pour the juice into them that will tend to prolong the life of the juice.

2. Fill the juice to the brim of the container. If there isn't enough juice, fill it up with clean boiled water. Make sure you do not leave any room for air because air contains oxygen, which reacts with the minerals of the juices and causes them to oxidize. It is, therefore, experts recommend the use of air tight jars.

3. Add in a bit of lemon juice to your prepared juice. This acts as a natural preservative and delays the oxidation process.

4. Keep away in the fridge and try to consume within 24 hours. A freezer will degrade the quality of the juice so unless it is necessary, do not freeze it. If you do have to, store it in ice-cube trays or plastic jugs and consume immediately after being defrosted.

Preparing juice is very easy and fun to do, storing juice too is really simple, but you have to be very careful with the whole process and do so only if necessary. It is best to consume the juice straight away, but for convenience sake, we've given tips and tricks to help you out with the whole diet process smoothly.

Homemade fresh juice is the best. Commercially available juices cannot match the quality of homemade juices fresh out of the juicer within seconds at any cost. Whenever you treat yourself to a glass of freshly made juice, drink it immediately. Please do not leave you juice too long in the refrigerator. You could have avoided the wastage by not preparing so much juice in the first place. Now that you have this extra juice left, it is a better option to discard it rather than sip it down to avoid wastage.

Drinking a glass of pre-prepared stale juice or consuming it unintentionally or by mistake can give you diarrhea or other diseases.

Chapter 8: Diet Plan for Weight Loss

These days our diets include more meat and fewer vegetables and fruits. The only ways we consume some fruits are either in the form of desserts or sweet juices. Vegetables, on the other hand, are very rarely eaten in the form of salads.

Now having known now all the advantages associated with the fresh fruits and vegetables, shouldn't we increase our intake of fruits and vegetables. If you're trying to lose weight, it's necessary to consume the right nutrients and eat and drink food that makes you feel full and satiated.

Vegetables Are Best For Shedding Pounds

Some of the best vegetables to help speed up weight loss are spinach, chard, lettuce, broccoli, kale, Brussels sprouts, turnips, asparagus, watercress, cauliflower, cabbage, tomatoes, carrots, peppers, parsnips, beans, beet root, celery, cucumbers and other leafy greens. These are rich in fiber, vitamins such as C, E and B, minerals such as chromium, magnesium and zinc all of which aid in speeding up metabolism and hence weight loss. A good combination of all these in your juice diet can provide nutrients that will enhance your capability to lose weight.

Juices for Weight Loss

You will find a number of juice recipes in various books and all over the internet that is said to be good for weight loss. All of these are made by including a combination of one or more of the vegetables above, some fruits along with some spices and herbs to enhance flavor and the capability to lose weight quickly. If you ask for one specific recipe of juice to lose weight, we are afraid there is not just one of it. There are loads of them. You have to try to find out which ones suit you best and whether you like them or not.

Vegetables used in juicing are more or less from the list given above. Fruits include apples, grapes, pineapples, cranberries, cherries, grapefruits, peaches, strawberries and watermelons among others.

Among herbs often parsley basil, mint, thyme etc. are used to bring flavor and additional vitamins to the juice. Cayenne peppers, garlic and ginger are used to bring additional goodness to the juice with their properties that aid in digestion.

Eating and Drinking Enough

With juices, the general recommendation is consuming about 32-64oz along with 6-8 glasses of water each day. It is okay to drink more, not fruit juices though. The more vegetable (or combination of vegetable and fruit juices) juices you drink the better. If you still feel hungry or thirsty, try drinking more water instead. Too little of anything is just as bad as too much as you harm yourself by not giving your body enough. The lack of nutrients will lead to starvation and diseases. Do not overeat as that may lead to weight gain and your ultimate goal of losing weight ends up in smoke.

It is really important to maintain a good balance between not eating and drinking too much or little. It is sort of very tricky because the definition of 'too much' or 'too little' varies from individual to individual. If you are not sure about the right quantities for yourself, it is best to consult your nutritionist, personal trainer or dietitian to ask what amounts of food and drink are suitable for you. They may vary from person to person based on their physical height and weight so make sure you know the right amount for you before you start your diet, or you can do yourself harm instead of good.

Going Off the Diet on a Bad Day

During the diet, you may feel a bit down, depressed or perhaps weak or sometimes events may occur such as a death in family or a break up in relationship, which makes you feel worse. What should you do on such days? Most of you wouldn't like to continue with the diet when you feel so upset, isn't it? Then, you ask yourself 'Is it okay to go off my diet for one day?'

The answer to this question given by different experts varies. In some cases, you can't help yourself such as in case of a death in family, and you do have to go off your diet. A day's cheat is fine for such cases, but any more than that, and your body starts going back to the same routine as before accepting more calories easily and adding fat cells to your body.

Some experts think this helps metabolism because your body isn't used to taking in many calories, and if you take them in on a day, it increases your metabolism to burn them away quickly. On the other hand, some experts disagree. They say if you do so once on a strict diet, you will want to do it again and again, and you can ruin your diet plan completely. Bingeing and not resisting to your cravings can be bad for weight loss regime.

Having Red Meat during the Diet

Most diet plans are around eating fresh fruits, vegetables and white meat such as poultry and seafood. Red meat and oily stuff are usually avoided in most of these. If you are a meat-lover, it could be difficult for you to give up meat during the diet. You may think having one portion of lean red meat during the entire day of every two to three days should be okay, but it won't do you much good. You can get the protein of the meat through beans, lentils or poultry and seafood so you don't really need red meat at all. Why not substitute something for a better form of protein. Of course, you compromise on the flavor and taste, but think about the good it will do you and after-effects of it. After all, it is just a matter of few days, and then you can have your regular meals in appropriate portions once you've achieved your weight loss target.

Do I need a Formal Diet Program When I have Difficulty Losing Weight?

As we mentioned earlier that not everybody lose weight quickly and easily. If you are one of those, you might be thinking about going on a formal diet program.

First, you need to find out why you're not losing weight. Is it your metabolism and your genetics or is it your carelessness? You can't do anything about your genetics, but can control your metabolism by consuming foods that are meant to increase metabolism and by exercising and doing a bit of work out. However, if you're being careless by not controlling your diet, eating too much, not getting enough sleep or not exercising then, we'd recommend consulting a personal trainer that would lead you on to a strict formal diet program to follow in order to lose weight. They will prepare a complete plan for you explaining what you should be eating and drinking during each day throughout the diet and what exercises to do at the same time.

Some people need somebody to guide them, or they simply won't do anything until and unless they are pressured to do so. For such people going on a formal diet is an excellent way because then they don't have to make a plan for themselves, but follow what they're being asked to do. If you're one of those don't hesitate to contact your personal trainer or dietitian who is there to guide and support people like you.

Chapter 9: Juicing and Exercise for Weight Loss

Juicing is an effective way to lose weight. However, exercising along with juicing can make your metabolism even better, and you are more likely to lose a lot of weight over a short period of time. There is no boundary on what exercises you should be doing. There is no such thing as the best exercise. As long as you are comfortable with it, find it enjoyable and can do it easily, it is the best exercise for you. It does not necessarily have to be a hard and strenuous exercise either. You can choose to do whatever you like.

Here are a few easy exercises discussed that can be used along with juicing to make weight loss an easier target to achieve over a very short period of time.

Walking

Walking is the easiest yet perhaps one of the best ways to exercise. It is not like walking from one aisle to another when you are shopping. You need a clear pathway or park or an area when you can walk continuously at a faster pace than you normally do. Walking for 30-60 minutes daily for 5-6 days a week speeds up your metabolic rate helping you lose weight faster. The number of calories you can lose through walking is dependent upon three factors:

- Your weight
- Your walking distance
- Walking pace

A rule of thumb is 100 calories per mile for a 180-pound person but it can vary depending on how fast you walk or whether you walk on a straight or steep road.

Running

Running is an extremely efficient yet an easy exercise that can help you shed off the extra pounds and get in good shape. Typically, a 150-pound person can lose approximately 100 calories per mile just by running. Run regularly, about 5-6 days a week approximately for one hour daily. Make it challenging for yourself. You can start by running 15 minutes every day for a week and gradually increase 5-10 minutes every week or so until you build enough stamina to run up one hour easily. It is important though that you do not wear yourself out. Run only as much as you can and keep yourself well-hydrated during the course.

Swimming

Swimming is a wonderful way to tone up and slim down because when you swim, you use all the major muscles of your body. It is easy to start with. If you can't swim, you can find a local pool where they provide classes for adults. Once you do that gradually start swimming one length and then increase to more, building your pace as you progress.

Swimming puts little stress on your body, and it is fun and relaxing at the same time. It also gives your cardiovascular system a great deal of workouts.

The best thing about swimming as an exercise is that you can tailor your swimming sessions to suit your needs. Typically, you can burn up to 550 calories in a half-hour session, but this can vary depending on your weight and the amount of effort you put in.

Yoga

Yoga doesn't increase your heartbeat and metabolism like other cardio exercises we talked about previously, but is a useful way to relax and keep stress at bay. Stress, as we discussed earlier, can lead to weight gain. So if during your diet you discover, you are not losing weight because of stress, yoga is a very helpful solution. It helps you mediate, make your body flexible and give you some time to relax without having to worry about all the miserable things going around in the world and perhaps in your life.

Other Cardio Exercises

Other than walking, running and swimming, there are several other cardio exercises that you can use along with your diet to enhance weight loss. They can give you a great deal of work out and can be adapted as a hobby too. You can do whichever you find easy and fun to do. Some of these are:

- Skiing
- Bicycling
- Rowing
- Aerobics

All of these are excellent ways to tone up and lose weight. There are other forms of exercise you can choose from. If you join a gym, you can have grouped exercises that are fun to do and easy because you have so many people with you doing the same. Also, you can have personal training sessions, which are specifically tailored to suit your needs.

How Much Should I Exercise for Weight Loss?

This is one common question that immediately comes to our minds, as soon as we talk about exercising. Generally, experts recommend exercising 4-5 days a week and between 30-60 minutes daily. If you can do more than that, that's fine as long as you are still active and are not overdoing it because you want to lose weight fast.

Losing weight takes time and a proper diet and exercise are tools that aid in weight loss. You cannot exactly determine how much weight you can lose over a fixed period of time. This is different for every person. However, if you follow the recommendation of exercising that is 4-5 days a week and between half-hour to one hour daily you will notice a clear difference in not only your weight and shape, but you will also start noticing just how you start to feel good about yourself.

Chapter 10: Setting Your Goal for Weight Loss Solution

Being Realistic at Setting Goals

Okay it is good to be realistic at setting goals. By realistic we mean thinking about an achievable target. For instance, for losing weight you might set a goal of losing one pound each week for three weeks by juice fasting. That is possible and is a fairly achievable target if you get everything right.

Compromises Made during the Diet and Being Prepared for them

There may be certain compromises that you may have to make during the whole process.

1. Discarding the Most Loved Clothes

Okay, this may be hard for some of you, but once you lose weight; the old clothes will no longer fit you. They will be big and very lose, and you will look like a skeleton wrapped up in huge sheets of clothing if you wear these. You do not want to look that way, do you? So start thinking about it now if you're prepared to lose them. We are aware that for most of you this shouldn't be a problem and will be something that will enchant them, but some people are too possessive about their old possessions and simply don't want them to go. This is meant for them. Ask yourself if you're ready to throw away clothes that are too big and no longer fit you.

2. Eating Differently from the Rest of the Members of Family

Of course when you are on a diet, you are eating completely different meals as compared to the rest of your family members, unless of course if you live all by yourself. This can give rise to conflicts; you may get lack of support and cooperation from others. Sometimes it may hurt their feelings even, for example; your mom can get hurt because you refuse to try her something special that she made specifically for you or when you are not having your meals with the rest of the family, others don't normally appreciate the idea at all.

You have to be prepared for this and explain to everybody in advance what you are trying to do and how this may affect your family life. If everybody in your house is mentally prepared for what is coming ahead this would avoid any conflicts during the diet. This is useful to do in advance so that you do not undergo any stress during the diet because of this reason.

3. Losing Weight: Pleasurable or Not?

To start with, a weight-loss program may sound fun and exciting, but it isn't for all. Not getting to eat what you want to and exercising that would bring pain to your muscles isn't quite pleasurable. These two things put off certain people from dieting completely. However, if you're prepared in advance about what is coming ahead, things become a lot easier.

You may find it pleasurable if you think of the after effects and you get support from friends and/or family.

4. Giving up Use of Cosmetics and Skincare Products
Very often in certain diet programs you are asked to refrain from the use of chemicals on your face and skin. This includes certain cosmetics and skin-care products. If you are a woman who is obsessed with her make-up and feel naked going out without it, this could be really hard for you.

Of course, you won't be asked to give up on the use all of your make-up and there is a strong chance that you would be allowed the use of everything, but you need to know that such a thing could happen. On a detox diet, for example, you aim to clarify your body from toxins so topical application of chemicals can make things worse. If you're asked to stop using any makeup while on a detox diet, it is definitely for your own good. Think about the after-effects of the diet: a clearer, fresher and younger-looking skin that wouldn't even need any makeup to disguise the acne and spots. That would be wonderful. Isn't it? So why worry if we cannot use our cosmetics for a few days' time. We may never need them again!

Again if you are prepared for this in advance, this should not be a big deal at all.

5. Making Health and Weight Control Top Priorities in Daily Life
No matter what type of diet plan you follow, your health and diet have to become your top-most priority if you really want to see a visible change in your weight, shape and size. Your mind has to set this goal to achieve a significant weight loss and bring you back in shape. All other things then come second.

Chapter 11: Ending Your Juice Fast Properly

Finally, we are towards the end of this report. We have explained juicing and weight loss both in an extremely detailed and easy manner so that when you start your juicing diet, you know exactly what you're doing, the benefits you can get out of it, it's possible symptoms and effective ways to shed off pounds using this method.

One thing that still remains to be discussed is how to end your juice fast properly. We'll throw some light on this topic in this very chapter. This is important to know because we cannot afford to give our bodies a sudden shock. Like when we started our juicing diet, we had to control our diet a few weeks before and gradually switched from solids to liquids; we need to do exactly the opposite of it when we move back from liquids to solids. The process had to be slow, starting new things each day so that our bodies can easily accept the new types of food we introduce it to after a certain period of time.

If you do not do end your juice diet properly by starting to eat solids straight away, you might start feeling sick and have digestion problems, which is not a very good idea. You definitely do not want to feel sick and have other problems after coming off a diet. You can start breaking your fast your way, but as a guideline we will explain here how to switch slowly. Within a week's time normally you can return to your regular food. If you want it to be slower, you can take two weeks. It is all up to you as long as it is safe and convenient to do so. We would generally suggest giving at least a week's time for your body before you return to solids such as red meat.

A Simple Sequence to Break Your Juice Fast in One Week

1st Day
Have your juice not more than twice a day. Eat raw fruits such as apples and leafy green vegetables for the rest of the day.

2nd Day
Have boiled or steamed vegetables for your meals with little or no seasoning. Consider having vegetables that are not too rich in starch such as spinach. Avoid having potatoes for the time being. Drink just one glass of juice either for breakfast, lunch or dinner.

3rd Day
You can start giving yourself a bit of starch now. The best thing to start with is brown rice. Cook the rice until really soft and chew it well so that your digestive system doesn't have to work too hard to digest it. Continue having raw fruits and salads on this day.

4th Day
Now you can start having a bit of dairy such as skimmed milk and yogurt. To give yourself some protein, having eggs on the fourth day is a really good idea.
5th Day
Now is the time to eat white meat such as poultry and fish. You can also have other seafood items if you like. You can have a bit more of starch such as in the form of bread or pasta.

6th Day:
Finally today is the day when you can start having your long-awaited 'red meat'. That's right! You can have lamb and beef if you like, but to start with have lean meat that is not overcooked and over spiced. You can have it with steamed vegetables and beans.

7th Day

From today onwards, you can eat anything you like, but be careful of eating because you do not want to let go all the effort you just made to get slimmer.

Eating and Drinking Normally

After seven days, you can start eating and drinking everything normally just like you used to, but in smaller portions so that you maintain your weight. You can enjoy your favorite foods, drinks and sweets, but all within limits. You can enjoy going out dine with family and friends as well. The best thing to do when you go and dine out is to order food in children's size portions or go for just the main and side and skip the dessert.

Go for a run, walk or jog 4-5 times a week and enjoy your normal routine life like you used to. No more compromises to make or hardships to go through. Everything will be just the same. What will change of course will be your weight and the way you look at food and consume it.

Chapter 12: Juice Diet Recipes for Weight Loss

Grapeberry Tonic

This delicious fruit mix is a nutritious way to lose weight. It is loaded with vitamins and minerals to cleanse the body and remove toxins and free radicals.

Ingredients:

2 cups grapes
2-3 cups strawberries

3 apricots
3 sprigs fresh mint

Procedure:

1.   Combine all ingredients together in the juicer.
2.   Fill each glass with ice cubes and pour juice over the top, stir
        and serve.

Makes 2 servings

Mediterranean Tonic Juice

Lose weight the vegetarian way! These vegetables are rich sources of
iron along with other vitamins and minerals.

Ingredients:

100g parsley
1-2 red pepper
1-2 cups broccoli florets
4 medium carrots

Procedure:

1.   Put ingredients through juicer in the same order as the list.
        Add flavor in the mix with lemon and orange juice if desired.
2.   Fill each glass with ice cubes and pour juice over the top, stir
        and serve

Makes 2 servings

Tonic Alkaline Juice

Drinking alkalizing fruits and vegetables can effectively tone excess fat
in the body.

Ingredients:

1 cucumber, peeled

3 stalks of celery
1 ½ Large handfuls of turnip greens
3 cloves of garlic peeled
Juice of ½ lemon

Procedure:

1.   Push all through the juicer.   Juice the greens by pushing
        them down with the cucumber or celery.
2.   Fill each glass with ice cubes and pour juice over the top, stir
        thoroughly until smooth and creamy.

Makes 2 servings

Watermelonics

This juice combination is a rich source of anti-oxidants such as vitamin C, beta-carotene and lutein which acts as protective scavengers against harmful free radicals that play a role in anti-aging and weight loss.

Ingredients:

1 ½ cup chunks of watermelon
2 medium cucumbers
1 cup mint leaves
1 cup chunk pineapple
2 medium eggplants

Procedure:

1.   Wash and peel the cucumbers and eggplants.
2.   Run all ingredients through the juicer.
3.   Fill each glass with ice cubes and pour juice over the top.
4.   Stir thoroughly until smooth and creamy.

Makes 2 servings.

Banberry Tonic

This is a delicious energy-booster drink rich in dietary fiber, vitamins, and minerals and packed with numerous health-promoting phytochemicals that ensure protection against diseases and cancers. A nutritious way to lose weight indeed!

Ingredients:

Juice of two oranges
2 bananas, peeled
½ cup fresh or frozen blueberries
½ cup fresh or frozen strawberries
1 ½ cup fresh rhubarb
1 ½ tsp. of honey

Procedure:

1.   Peel oranges and bananas.
2.   Place ingredients in juicer and process until frothy and smooth.
3.   Fill each glass with ice cubes and pour juice over the top.

Makes 2 servings drink and enjoy!

Applelicious Slender Drink

This drink is a nutritious way to lose weight. Apples are low in calories, but contain good quantities of vitamin-C and beta-carotene, which is a powerful natural antioxidant and helps the body develop resistance against infectious diseases. Vegetables are also loaded with antioxidants that protect the body from oxidant stress and cancers, as well as help boosts the immune system.

Ingredients:

2 ½ cups grated apple
2 ½ cups finely grated pear
¼ cup raisins
½ cup spinach
1 ½ tbsp. ground almonds

2 bananas, peeled
Cinnamon to taste

Procedure:

1.   Wash the stuff, cut into small sections if needed.
1.   Juice the apples and set aside. Juice all the remaining ingredients.
2.   Fill each glass with ice cubes and pour juice over the top.
3.   Add the apple juice, sprinkle with ground almonds and cinnamon. Stir and enjoy.

Makes 2 servings

Coco Reducer Delight

Coconut, banana and spinach all contain the electrolyte potassium that help maintain fluid balance; promote proper metabolism and muscle function and help maintain proper function of kidney and bladder. The coconut meat contains lauric acid, which is beneficial in fighting off infections. This slimming juice can provide an excellent amount of calcium, folic acid, vitamin K, lutein, and iron.

Ingredients:

1 cup shredded coconut meat
2 large apples
2 large bananas
1 tbsp. chopped spinach
1 tbsp. currant
¼ cup ground almonds or sunflower seeds
½ tsp. cinnamon to taste

Procedure:

1.   Run all ingredients through a juicer.
2.   Fill each glass with ice cubes and pour juice over the top.
3.   Mix well, sprinkle with ground almonds and cinnamon.

Makes 2 servings

Fit & Loss Drink

Spinach is one of the vegetables recommended in cholesterol controlling and weight reduction. This vegetable and fruit juice combination is a very rich source of heart-healthy electrolytes, antioxidant, vitamins and minerals that gives the body energy and immunity resistance against infectious diseases.

Ingredients:

½ cup spinach
½ cup dried figs
½ cup dried apricots
2 bananas
1 kiwi
1 pear
8 strawberries

Procedure:

1.   Rehydrate dried fruits in 2 cups of water overnight or for several hours.
2.   Put all ingredients together in the juicer.
3.   Fill each glass with ice cube and pour juice over the top. Stir thoroughly until smooth.

Makes 3 servings drink and enjoy!

Tinny Shaky Delight

This juice blend is a good source of anti-oxidants and dietary fiber for protection against certain types of cancer. Drinking this juice regularly helps prevent osteoporosis, relieve constipation and help the body develop resistance against infectious diseases.

Ingredients:

2 large Fuji apples
2 tbsp. raisins

Juice of one orange
½ cucumber
½ tbsp. chopped green cabbage
1 tbsp. maple syrup
¼ tsp. cinnamon to taste
Dash nutmeg to taste
Dash cardamom to taste

Procedure:

1.   Wash fruits and vegetables.   Cut to the size that will fit in your juicer.   Push the raw foods through the juicer machine.
2.   Fill each glass with ice cubes and pour juice over the top.
3.   Sprinkle with dash nutmeg, cardamom and cinnamon.   Stir thoroughly until smooth.

Makes 2 serving drink and enjoy!

Light Celery Tonic

Celery and cucumber are low-calorie vegetables but rich sources of dietary fiber, an ideal combination for weight loss. This is a refreshing mix of fruits and vegetables, which are all rich in vitamins and anti-oxidants.   This cooler can help reduce inflammation and give protection against cancer.

Ingredients:

1 cup chopped stalk celery
½ cucumber, peeled
2 bananas, peeled
2 apples, sliced
2 medium carrots
Juice of one lemon
3 tbsp. soaked raisins
1 tbsp. finely ground almonds or pecans (optional)

Procedure:

1. Wash all the ingredients. Run them through a juicer. Take the expelled pulp and run it back through the juicer a second time to extract all liquid.
2. Fill each glass with ice cubes and pour juice over the top.
3. Sprinkle with ground almonds.
4. Stir juice and serve immediately for the greatest nutritional benefit.

Makes 1 to 2 servings

Quick Slimmer

This is a low-calorie juice drink which can help strengthen the bones, and loaded with anti-oxidants to help keep your body healthy. Try this innovative juice drink tonic and see how energetic and alive you feel the following day.

Ingredients:

1 head romaine lettuce
1 head cauliflower
Juice of one lemon
1 apple
1 avocado
2 tomatoes
1 red onion
1 cup sprouts
¼ tsp. chili powder or dash of cayenne

Procedure:

1. Wash all veggies and run them through the juicer. Run the pulp back through the juicer a second time.
2. Mash avocado and combine with remaining ingredients.
3. Fill each glass with ice cubes and pour juice over the top.
4. Stir thoroughly until smooth and creamy. Serve and enjoy.

Makes 2 to 3 servings

Slim Kiwi Tonic

This juice blend is rich in fiber and flavonoids that help lower body cholesterol level and improve blood flow. This is also an excellent source of anti-oxidant vitamins A, C and E as well as B-complex and beta carotene that boosts the immune system and protects the body against harmful free radicals.

Ingredients:

2 kiwis, peeled
2 pears
1 medium cucumber
1 avocado
½ orange
½ cup sunflower or alfalfa sprouts

Procedure:

1.   Wash all ingredients and run them through the juicer.
2.   Mash avocado and combine with remaining ingredients.
3.   Fill each glass with ice cubes and pour juice over the top.
4.   Stir thoroughly until smooth and creamy. Serve and enjoy.

Makes 2 servings

Sprout Tonic

This juice blend is an excellent source of vitamin C, which is necessary to make and maintain collagen, the connective tissue that holds body cells together. It also helps build teeth and bones, strengthens the walls of capillaries and other blood vessels, as well as promotes healing of wounds and burns. This juice drink also helps the body neutralize carcinogens by protecting its ability to recognize and eliminate malignant cells.

Ingredients:

3 cups mung bean sprouts
4 apples
1 cup bokchoy or Chinese cabbage
2 turnip roots
½ cup tahini

Procedure:

1. Wash veggies, fruits and run them through the juicer. Put all ingredients together in the juicer.
2. Fill each glass with ice cubes and pour juice over the top.
3. Stir juice and serve immediately for the greatest nutritional benefit.

Makes 1 to 2 servings

Fit & Shape Tonic

This juice blend is loaded with dietary fiber and vitamins A and C, folate, potassium and lycopene, which help increase bulk of the food by absorbing water throughout the digestive system and helps in easing constipation, treat gout, high blood pressure and protect against some cancers.

Ingredients:

Juice of one lemon
1 medium tomato
4 stalks celery
½ clove garlic or ¼ onion
½ cup tahini
½ tsp. thyme, basil
Dash of cayenne pepper

Procedure:

1. Wash veggies and fruits thoroughly. Put together in the juicer.
2. Fill each glass with ice cubes and pour juice over the top.
3. Stir thoroughly until smooth and creamy.

Makes 1 to 2 servings

Slimmix Juice

This vegetable mix is a good source of anti-oxidant vitamins A, C, E and K, as well as potassium, manganese, zinc and flavonoids that help block cancer-causing substances and bolster immunity. This is an excellent source of beta carotene, a nutrient that is essential for healthy hair, skin, eyes, bones and mucous membranes.

Ingredients:

4 cups chopped spinach
2 medium tomatoes
2 cups sliced zucchini
2 medium carrots
1 cup alfalfa sprouts
1/3 cup feta cheese (optional)
2 tbsp. minced cilantro or basil
½ lemon juice
1 tbsp. honey

Procedure:

1.   Wash all veggies and run them through the juicer.
2.   Combine remaining ingredients.
3.   Fill each glass with ice cubes and pour juice over the top.
4.   Stir thoroughly until smooth and creamy.

Makes 2 servings, drink and enjoy!

Tasty Willowy Juice

This juice blend contains lycopene, compounds that can lessen the cancer-causing potential of estrogen and induce production of enzymes that protect against diseases.   This juice is a rich source of vitamin A, C, potassium and beta carotene, which are beneficial for the heart and help in lowering the cholesterol level.

Ingredients:

4 large carrots
2 large stalks celery
7 large kale leaves
Handful of romaine leaves
Handful of parsley
½ small beet
2 tomatoes
1 red bell pepper
½ cucumber
2 cups alfalfa, clover, or sunflower sprouts
Optional: 2 cloves garlic, dash of cayenne

Procedure:

1. Wash all ingredients and run them through the juicer. Run the pulp back through the juicer a second time.
2. Fill each glass with ice cubes and pour juice over the top.
3. Stir thoroughly until smooth and creamy. Serve and enjoy.
4. Makes 2 to 3 servings

Thirsty Tonic

This juice is rich in electrolytes and water content that can beat tropical summer thirst. This juice combination is an excellent source of Vitamin A, C, folate, potassium and iron as well as pectin that helps control blood cholesterol levels and essential for vision and immunity. It added mint taste helps relieve fatigue and stress.

Ingredients:

½ watermelon
½ cantaloupe peeled
1 pear
Juice of one lemon
1 handful mint

Procedure:

1.   Wash all ingredients and run them through the juicer.
2.   Fill each glass with ice cube and pour juice over the top. Stir thoroughly until smooth.

Makes 1 to 2 servings

Drink and enjoy!

Flimsy Juice

Low in calories, but a good source of energy boosting vitamins, this juice drink is recommended for those who want to reduce weight quickly. This juice is high in fiber, including the soluble type that lowers elevated blood cholesterol levels.

Ingredients:

½ head red cabbage
1 zucchini
1 red onion
Juice of one lemon
1 cup chopped of parsley
1 cup toasted sesame seeds

Procedure:

1.   Push all ingredients through the juicer.
2.   Fill each glass with ice cubes and pour juice over the top. Stir thoroughly until smooth.

Makes 2 servings.

Drink and enjoy!

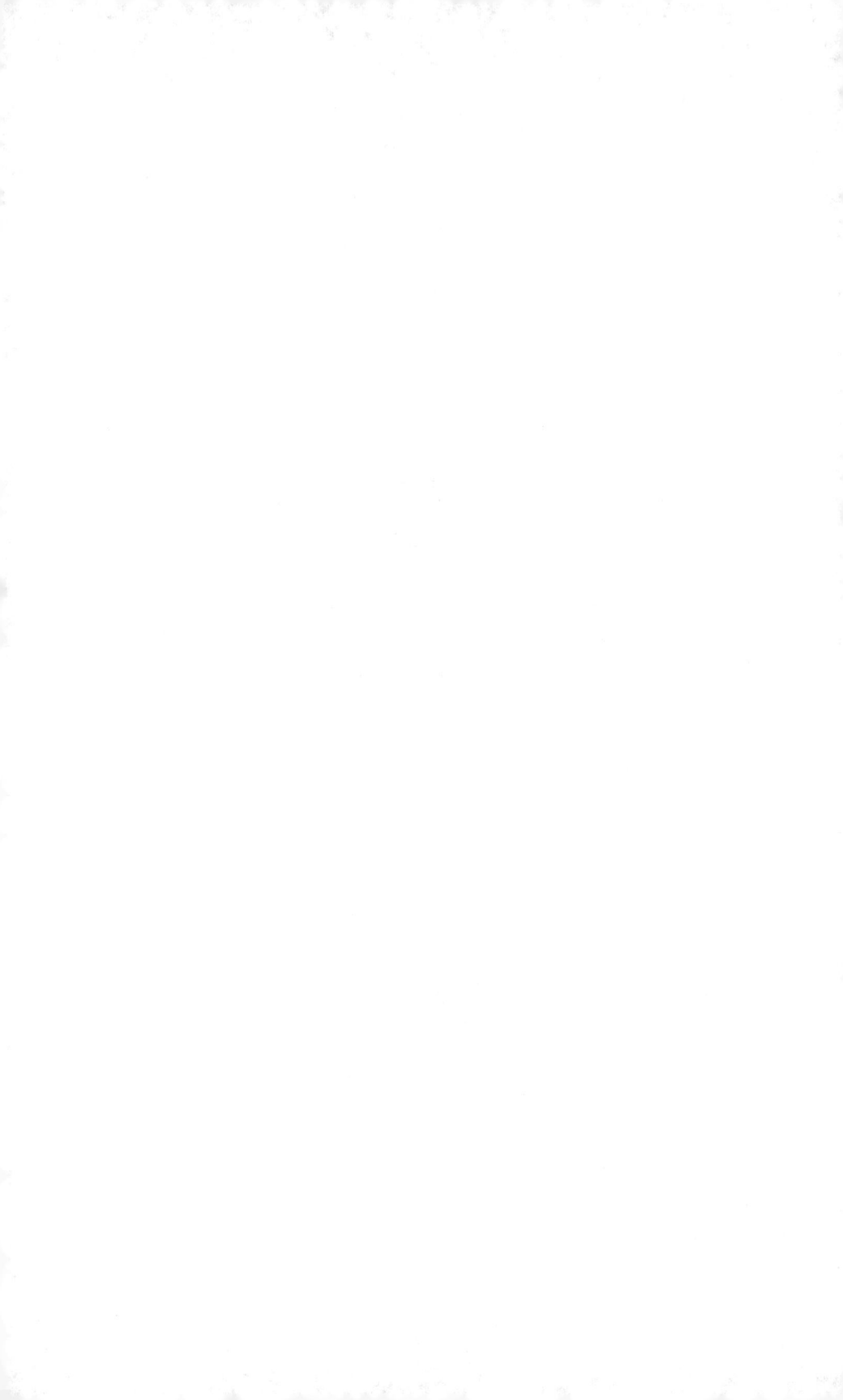

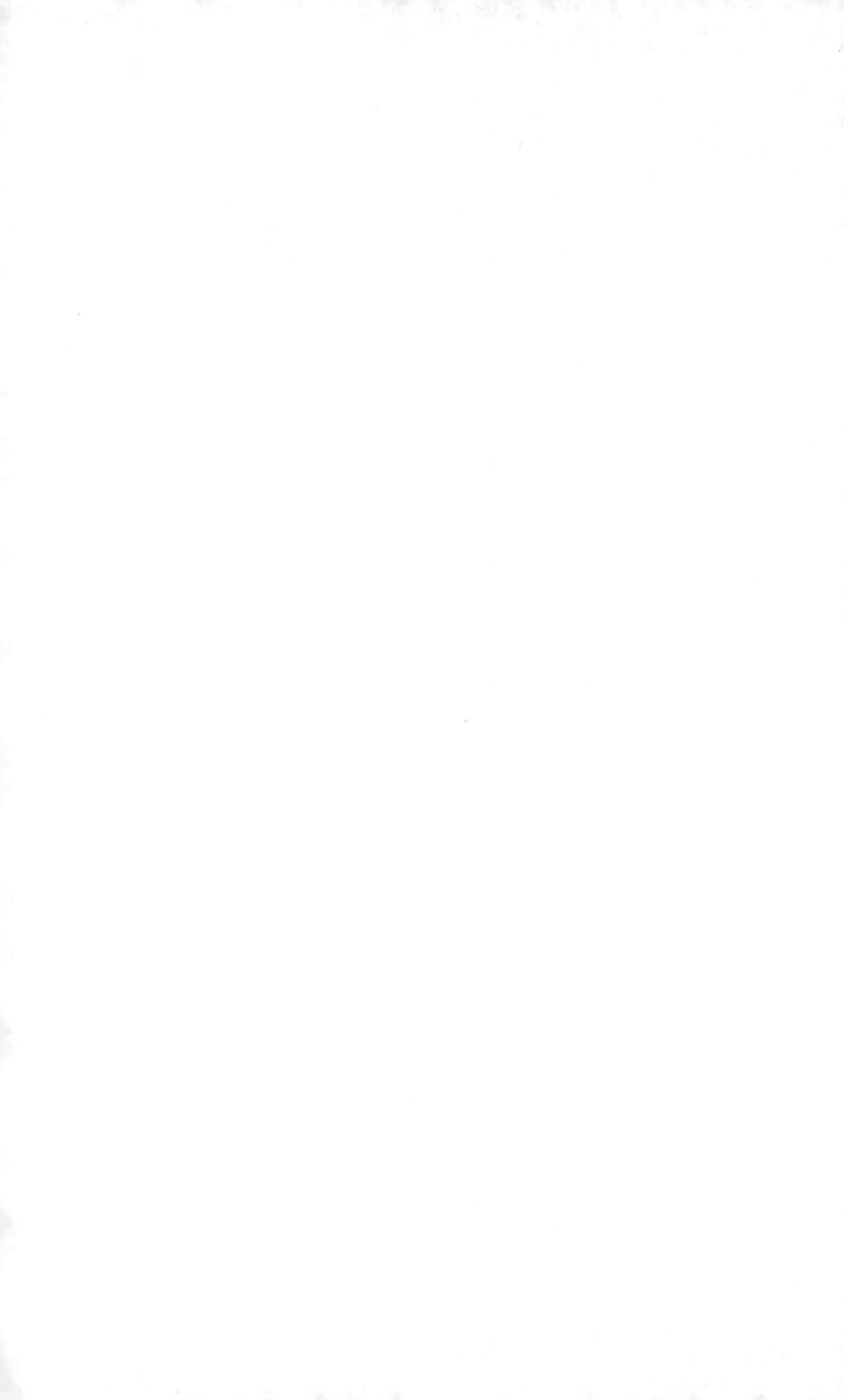

www.ingramcontent.com/pod-product-compliance
Lightning Source LLC
Chambersburg PA
CBHW070348300526
45791CB00023B/1156